"Begin with the end in mind."

-Stephen R. Covey

I wrote this this book to highlight the importance of communications in nursing as it relates to patient perception to receiving quality care. The problem that many hospitals face is that they are delivering high-quality care, but they are getting marginal or lackluster reviews from their patients. This book provides some of the guiding principles nurses can utilize during the course of their duties. By doing so, any nurse can have impactful patient interactions, provide psychosocial therapeutic dialogue, and ultimately get their hospital the recognition it deserves. Consequently, the patient's answers to hospital surveys will accurately reflect the good work that the nurses do.

I have tailored this book for the nursing administration, registered nurses, licensed practical nurses, and nursing assistants. However, this book and the principles discussed are also applicable to help medical doctors improve their notorious reputation for having a horrible bedside manner. Finally, this book is for anyone who wants to improve their communication skills, as these principles are applica-

ble in all disciplines, occupations, and relationships.

After you complete this book and
begin to apply these principles, I can promise you that you will notice an unquanti-
fiable, positive change in your interactions
with your patients, your co-workers, and in
your personal relationships. You will find
your self-esteem improving. When you begin disciplining your efforts to improve
communication, you will not only help to
improve the hospital's survey scores, but
your life. Helping you improve your life
and bring you more joy is the true inten-
tion of this book.

Chapter One

What Is Nursing Communication?

"The most important thing in communication is hearing what isn't said."

-Peter F. Drucker

I once had a patient who was a young black man in his late 20's. He had this rare condition where he had boil-like cysts that were very painful and gave off a bad odor. This young male patient had Hidradenitis Suppurativa and he had abscesses throughout his body. They were on his back, his buttocks, his groin, his arms, his neck, and his legs. Besides the foul smell, they caused him tremendous pain to the extent that he couldn't sit up or lay down.

It was affecting his relationship with his girlfriend, his son, going out in public, and being out with his family. The doctors were reluctant to give him morphine, which would help assuage his pain situation. Even though his primary doctor recommended morphine for the pain, the hospital doctors hesitated because they were thinking that he might be someone who was simply drug seeking.

With my expertise and background, my gut was telling me that this person wasn't really drug seeking, but he was in actual pain and that I should listen to him. I took the time to sit down and do just that. I gave him all the time in the world necessary, adjusted my body language accordingly, made eye contact, and really helped him to understand and open up. He cried several times in that conversation and I received the details of how it was affecting the relationship with his son, sex between him and his girlfriend, and how he felt.

By giving me the details about the pain he was in, I was able to see what was truly going on with him. This therapeutic communication allowed me to advocate to the doctors on his behalf that he truly needed stronger pain medication. I suggested they sit down with him and further assess his pain level to see what they could do.

Through my efforts, the doctors came in a second time and spoke to him in more detail. After a lengthy conversation, they could see the depth of his pain and that it was genuine. They increased his pain medication, and sure enough, he did feel better. The patient was very grateful for me advocating for him. He appreciated that I took the time to listen to his story, understand him, and see his needs. We achieved a good rapport. This led to his satisfaction at the hospital greatly improving. He gave us wonderful ratings. In addition, he told my manager about the excellent care that I had given him, which made me feel good.

As that example illustrates, communication is the cornerstone of nursing. To understand what a patient feels by actively listening to them goes hand-in-hand with an astute nursing assessment. Furthermore, by putting yourself in their shoes, you can better relate to them and advocate on their behalf. This can make all the difference in their treatment and ability to get well.

My definition for nursing communication is an empathic, therapeutic, active listening that is patient-centered, and allows patients to verbalize his or her feelings. The key words here in this definition are "therapeutic," "active listening," and "patient centered." Let me break down each of these crucial words.

Therapeutic

A simple way to describe therapeutic is "feeling better." The goal is to make sure that the patient feels better during the conversation and at its conclusion. You achieve this by allowing the patient to verbalize his or her feelings. When the patient has the opportunity to do this, no matter how happy or how sad they are, do not turn around and make it about you. Many times when the patient gets sad, a nurse may try to walk away or minimize the patients affliction by say "everything is going to be alright" or other similar clichés.

Allow the patient to talk, even though they are feeling sad. By getting it off their chest and saying what they need to say, they will have a therapeutic benefit. They are given permission to not 'hold everything in'. If they continue to keep everything in, they are going to cause emotional damage to themselves. Consequently, increasing the difficulty to make intelligent and informed decisions about their healthcare.

Allowing a therapeutic environment in any conversation with a patient will enhance the patient's feeling that somebody cared. This is what the essence of nursing is truly about. Not just in doing the tasks the job calls for, but really showing that you care for the patient. You want the best for your patients. You recognize that you are not just there to administer medications, but to be there for them. As nurses, we are not just there for their physical well-being, but also their mental and emotional welfare. By creating this therapeutic environment, you will be helping a patient with all of these.

Active Listening

The key to active listening is to be totally involved with the conversation. Listening is not just a mental exercise, it is physical as well. You need to sit eye level with the patient. Your body language should mirror that of the patient. While it is important to make eye contact, you do need to be aware of their hand gestures and their overall body language. This shows your patient that you are intently focusing on them. Nothing else matters to you.

This is important because the patient needs this proof in order to understand that the nurse is actually listening. They know you are engaged in the conversation and that you care what they have to say. When the patient has that feeling, he or she is inclined to share more information. The patient will feel the benefits of the therapeutic communication and interaction.

Patient Centered

Like active listening, this shows the patient that you are focusing on them. You are not talking about how your day went, or how the patient's story connects back to yours. *It is not about you. It is about the patient.* They do not want to know how tired you are, or how short-staffed the unit is, or why you are not there to grant the patient's request. It is about keeping the patient focused in your mind. You need to be service-oriented towards the patient and doing everything you can for that person. By having that mental framework, you will keep the focus on the patient.

You want to understand how the patient feels through everything they say or do. You want them to understand their own feelings and help them with their issues. When the patient feels that everything that you do and say focuses on their total well-being, both physically and emotionally, it will have a drastic impact. They will be more willing to open up and to share. This will give you a deeper understanding to the root causes of the patient's emotions and lead to a more therapeutic experience for them.

Chapter Two

Love Your Patients

"Love begins at home. It's not how much we do, but how much love we put in that action." -Mother Theresa.

     I want to share another story with you. One time I admitted a 67-year-old affluent, lonely white man. He suffered from advanced COPD. He had a tracheostomy, diabetes, hypertension, CHF; the list seemed endless. He had a very childish and bratty behavior. When he did not get his way, he would raise a fit. He would also incessantly ring the call bell. He would even ring the bell when you were in his room talking with him. Then, just as you are about to walk out the door after you make sure you met all of his needs, he would ring it again. I believe it was because he was lonely and he wanted someone to always be there.

It seemed as if it might be part of a nervous tic or compulsion. Nevertheless, this made taking care of him very difficult and time consuming. If people did not respond quick enough, he would keep you in the room for 30 minutes at a time. This was dangerous for the other patients in our care. He would even take off his trach so that the alarm would sound. It did not matter to him that this impaired his ability to breathe even further with his COPD.

He became a very challenging patient. Once we had to call in rapid response because he kept taking off the trach and he was having difficulty breathing. I should mention that we had him for nine months. One moment he would be very nice and sweet, and the next moment he'd be very rude and frustrated. He was immobile, he had difficulty breathing, and he was very unhappy at times.

We all knew deep down that he did love and appreciate us. Many times his requests were on the line of, "Oh, move the juice a little bit to the left. Oh no, move it a little bit to the right. Oh, could you pass me the roll." These little requests were to keep us in the room so he would not feel lonely. After all these requests, he would look at you nicely and softly say, "Thank you." When it was finally time for him to be discharged, he would fight it. They called me in because they knew that I had established a very strong rapport with the man.

The staff asked me to see if I could talk to him and if I could influence him into making the decision to leave. After doing so, I got him to agree that it was time to leave. However, when the EMT people came into his room, he would change his mind again because he saw it was actually time for him to go. What we did was place him on the EMT stretcher anyway. Then he accepted his fate and the hospital could finally discharge him.

This is an extreme example, but I want to show that as nurses and medical professionals, there is an emotional component of love and caring for what we do. Nursing is caring and an element of love is to care for someone. My definition of love is wanting the best for somebody. We want the best for our patients. Even though we are professionals, we do love our patients.

"Love begins at home" is a true saying, but we could substitute the word "home" with "hospital" and say love begins at the hospital. It's not how much we do, but it's how much love we put into that action. We need to create our hospital as if it was our home, and treat the people in there as if they were our guests. We need to be very loving and put that love into every action that we do. This leads me to the top three ways to increase patient satisfaction.

Number one is communication, of course. This means good communication amongst everyone involved: doctors, nurses, patients, technicians, patients' families, etc. It needs to be present in everything from intake to discharge. When a patient is discharged, he or she needs to be crystal clear on follow-up, pain management, and any medications. Discharge procedures are very important for every hospital. It is a real test of communication between doctors and nurses. It is paramount that the communication between the healthcare professionals and the patients is sublime and nonpareil.

The second way to increase patient satisfaction is to be a nurse of your word. To rephrase it, be responsive to your patients while maintaining your integrity. As you see, a great deal of this is rooted in communication as well. You have to demonstrate integrity by doing for a patient what you said you would do. If you say you are going to be back in five minutes, be back in five minutes. Furthermore, be responsive. If you say you love your patients and want the best for them, you are going to want to minimize their suffering as much as possible. Be proactive in your assessments and interventions. There is no replacing effective and efficient care. A key component to increasing patient satisfaction is by being proactive in caring for the patient's needs, reducing suffering.

The third key to patient satisfaction is cleanliness. The nursefluential do their best to create a home-like environment in the hospital. It should not have the atmosphere of a foreign jail. If you can envision the hospital as being a second home, then you can see the importance of keeping that home clean. This shows respect for your environment and for your health. Cleanliness is a staple of nursing and of medicine. When the staff and the hospital care and respect the cleanliness of the unit, then the patients are going to feel as if the staff respects them. Subsequently, the patients will feel safe in their new environment. In addition, they are going to have a higher perceived value of the hospital and of their care.

We need to ensure that these three facets of patient satisfaction are at the forefront of our minds. It all starts with communication. Then, we need to back up whatever we say to a patient through our actions. Concomitantly, we have to demonstrate a true love and respect towards our environment. In turn, this helps patients perceive the love and respect the hospital staff has for its patients.

Chapter Three

Top Three Attitudes Patients Want in Their Nurse

"Your attitude, not your aptitude will determine your altitude."

-Zig Ziglar.

Here is a story about a situation I had with a patient. He was Hispanic and had many issues. His diagnosis included Hepatitis C, AIDS, liver failure, drug abuse, diabetes, ataxia...you name it, and he seemed to have it. He was a stubborn man in his late 30's or early 40's. He insisted on using the toilet instead of the commode, even though he was too weak to make the trip. In order to promote his functionality and his psychological well-being, we took him to the toilet and told him to ring the call bell when he was finished. When he rang the bell, I discovered that he had feces all over himself. His family complained about me and my nursing abilities, and any of staff that were present. I told them to please hold on so I could get some assistance. I told the patient, "Please stay in the toilet. Let me get some things so I can clean you up." I went to go get what I needed, but he had no patience. When I came back, he was standing up in the bathroom and trying to mobilize himself. He had feces all over the place.

I had to have two or three people assist me. While we were trying to get him cleaned up, his family was yelling at us, saying, "They don't know what they are doing. Look at this big black nurse; he doesn't know what he is talking about!" This added to the ruckus. I stayed unperturbed, full of equanimity, calm and relaxed. I understood that they were very frustrated, and their father was dying. They were just taking it out on me and the situation. I looked at is as a way to let them vent.

We were able to put him back in the bed, clean him up, and let the family know that we were there for them, and that was that. He ended up being discharged later, but, unfortunately, the family wasn't very happy with our care.

I had him as a patient again. I enjoyed having him. I didn't take anything personally so what he said did not bother me. I found him to be a kind soul, and I did my best to take care of him every time. On this occasion, his diabetes was very, very brittle. He ended up going into hypoglycemia at about a 20 blood sugar. We had to call rapid response, put some D-50 into him, and we successfully brought him back to baseline.

The patient woke up three hours later and I gave him a hamburger for lunch. He said, "This goddamn place serves these dry-ass hamburgers and shit with no ketchup. I can't believe this shit!"

I responded, "Sir, you do realize that you almost died today and we saved your life, right?"

He replied, "Really? What happened?" I then said, "Never mind, my man, I'll go find you some ketchup."

For me it was an honor to save his life, and I felt very happy to just be there and take care of him, even if he did not fully appreciate everything that we were doing. I still treated him with care, compassion, and love. He knew that, and he always looked forward to having me as his nurse. While his family still acted irate, he didn't.

He ended up being discharged again. However, about a week or two later,

I saw him arrive in the emergency room. I saluted him and his family, and they remembered me. They realized that I didn't take what they said in the past personally, and they treated me very cordially.

A few weeks later, I am going through the emergency room area to start my shift and I see his two daughters crying. Although they had been very bellicose with me in the past, I asked them, "What's going on? How is everything? How's your father? What can I do to support you?" They told me that he passed away and they were very sad. They each gave me hugs and I was able to console and be somewhat therapeutic to them. They ended up telling me that they were very happy with my care of their father and they apologized for their behavior. They explained they were going through a lot.

In conclusion, he was one of my most memorable patients. This story helps illustrate the key principles that I was able to use in the heat of the moment. Moreover, they are principles that I utilize all the time.

Understanding is the first of these concepts. By this, I mean having the attitude of understanding, wanting to understand, and to feel what they feel. You have to realize that how a patient acts towards you is never personal. It is a result of what they are going through. You have to have an attitude of service and of caring. When you operate from that perspective, it is easier to put your feelings aside and make it about them. Having this sense of under-standing is paramount. When you under-stand how a patient's emotions are at play when they are in a hospital, then you also comprehend his or her behaviors in the context of the situation. With understand-ing, you are able to easily transition into the next attitude.

The attitude of maintaining a solu-tion-orientated mindset is the second ma-jor attitude. To find solutions to our pa-tients' problems is the main reason why our hospitals exist. When you fully under-stand your patient's situation, then you can focus on the solution. Even if you are at fault as a nurse, don't dwell on the er-ror. One of my favorite phrases is, "I made a mistake, I'm sorry about that. What can

I do to make this right? What can I do to make it better?"

Always be in a solution-orientated mindset. One of my favorite quotes is, "If you bring a problem without a solution, then you're just complaining" - Robert Riopel. Complaining is not something that we want to do. We don't want to have a complaining mindset, which is negative. This perfectly leads into the third attitude, which is to stay positive and optimistic throughout any type of problem.

Many times as a nurse, we can face dire situations. The outlook is bleak and dismal, because the person is going to die. However, I always project a positive nature. I tell family members that this is really one of the most beautiful parts of somebody's life, the dying process. If we can, we are going to do everything in our power to let this person die with dignity and shower them with love. I let the family know that they can let their family member know that they made a difference, and that they as a family can make a difference in their loved one's dying process. I tell them that we all have to accept that we are each going to die. The following is one of my favorite explanations that I like to share with the family of my patient: "Think about it this way, if it was you in that bed, how would you want your family members to treat you? Would you want them to be crying all the time, or would you want them to be positive? Be loving and grateful, talk about the good old days while they are laying there."

While I know that they are going through a difficult, sad, and emotional time, I am able to bring share positive vantage point to help the family cope with the situation. By doing that, I am able to increase the satisfaction that the patients and family members have with my care.

I want to highlight the fact that even in a life and death situation, most people cannot see any good in it. You can make the best out of any situation by being totally in the moment by loving and caring for everybody there. Show them the value of reminiscing about the good times and loving the person leaving this world. By being obstinately positive, you can show them the good, the ray of hope that everyone would have missed. You can make the difference in every patient experience, whether its a joyous healthy birth of a newborn, or a bleak death of a loved one. Your positivity can, at the very least, make the experience more palatable for all those involved.

In brief, these three attitudes will have your patients requesting you to be their nurse. This is what you want. However, it is a process to master them, and it is not easy. Nonetheless, there are many benefits for doing so, not just with your patients, but also within yourself. The consequences of these actions are that you will find yourself being even more positive. You will improve your ability to find a solution in any situation. Most of all, you will establish a deeper understanding of yourself and of your connections with other people. You will also have more enriching relationships. This includes your relationship with your patients, which will help the patients' relationship with the hospital. You will also feel more satisfaction with your job, which will lead to a happier unit, which further creates a happier patient experience. Understanding, being solution-oriented, and being positive will foster improved patient satisfaction and will improve the perception of the hospital experience.

Chapter Four

Three Communication Principles to Have Your Patients Love You

"I am a great believer that any tool that enhances communication has profound effects in terms of how people can learn from each other and how they can achieve the kinds of freedom that they're interested in."

-Bill Gates.

Here is a story about an admission I had. A black man and his mother came in. The man seemed very distraught and upset. His mother was very ill, sick, and dying. When he saw me, another young, tall, black young man and saw that I was her nurse, it was a little bit outside of his paradigm. I saw his reaction, I could tell he was wondering whether I would be a good nurse. He already had a bad experience in the emergency room when he made a request of the emergency nurse. That person shrugged him off and said, "No. I'm busy right now." That person didn't take the time to fulfill a simple request of passing him more water and getting him a towel, and he was very upset. He told her that it was uncalled for. She ended up apologizing later, but this bad experience still bothered him. Now he was going to be in our care.

When I saw the situation, I could tell that he was concerned if I would be able to provide expert level care. What I did was use my first principle, which is 'keep it real' and sincere. I looked him in his eye, shook his hand, and I told him, "We here are the Hospice & Palliative Care Unit. I apologize for what had happened in the ER. Here on this unit, we take great pride and are experts in what we do. We are all here for a reason. We are passion- ate and I have lost my own mother. She was also a patient on one of these units, just as your mother is. That's the reason why I'm so passionate as a palliative care nurse." As I continued to look him in the eyes, I told him, "I am going to treat your mother as if she's my mother and your family as if you're my family. I'm going to do the best that I can to make sure she is comfortable during this very special process in her life."

With that, he relaxed and calmed down. He let out a deep breath and gave me a hug. He stopped asking the type of questions family members ask when they don't trust in your abilities as a healthcare professional. He was accustomed to asking question after question, just to make sure the hospital was on top of things. That came to a sudden halt when he met me. He told all of his family what a great nurse they had. Soon, all of his family knew me. When she did pass away after the next couple of days, I was able to give them all hugs, help them through their situation, and support them. They felt like they had a great experience.

The most important moral to the story above is the importance of being sincere. Other techniques that you learn from me will not be effective if you are not sincere. People are very intelligent, a lot more intelligent than you realize. Often, they can tell whether you are being authentic or full of garbage. Even if they don't have any proof, they can feel it, they will have a nagging sense of unease. You have to be sincere, you have to mean what you say. If you don't do that, then you are not going to be nursefluential.

That leads me to another key principle. You have to put yourself in their shoes. The word here is "empathy." You have to feel what they feel. When I told that man that my mother and I had the same situation, I was able to empathize with him. I was able to keep it real and let him know that I had a relevant story that would tie back to him. By empathizing with somebody, you have to do your best to feel what they feel and to actually feel the emotion. Think about what you would be doing in that situation. How you would want to be treated? What are your concerns? Let the emotions run through you and see what your reaction is for that emotion.

In my story, you can see that I saw his frustration and I understood where he was coming from. I was able to put myself in his shoes as a man who really wanted to make sure that his mother received the best care through her dying days. After he had a bad experience in the ER, he admitted that then he first saw me he wondered, "What could a male nurse who was younger than him do for his mother?" By me having that ability to be insightful and step outside of myself, I was able to calm him down and concentrate on the care his mother needed.

Again, an important point here is never take anything personal when you are at the job. Whatever a patient says or does is based on how they view and see the world. Once you take it personally, then that could lead to frustrations like the emergency nurse experienced. You cannot have the attitude of, "They're not respecting my time. Don't they see that I'm busy?!" Putting it in an impersonal sense, you would say, "Hey listen, if my mother was dying, it would be hard for me to be considerate to any other staff member at a hospital that's here to serve me and my family. All I really want to do is make sure that my mother is taken care of. If I could do it myself, I would, but I don't know how." The ER nurse finally apologized after that family member very gently and appropriately confronted her for her lack of communication. In the end she was able to get out of her own head and see that she was at fault. I am very proud to say that she was able to apologize.

This story is very relevant, because it leads us to the third major principle that really wraps it all up. The third major principle is to make others feel important. You want to show that you genuinely value them, whether you are dealing with the patient, family, or both. You believe that their thoughts, feelings, and beliefs are important. One of the major drives that we have as humans is to feel important. We want to believe that what we say, and what we do, make a difference.

When you arrive late or scoff at a request the patient's family makes, you are showing them that they are not impor- tant. This is especially true in a sensitive situation as when the mother is dying and the son makes a request to clean her lips with a wet towel. Even though it is not a life or death request, the key is that the son wants to feel that his mother's life is still important. He also wants to know that he is important and that his family is important to me. The nurse needs to recognize this and never forget it. I know we do get busy, but we cannot let ourselves and the importance of our job, cloud over the importance of the feelings of the patient and/or family. They have to be taken in to consideration.

These principles do not just apply to working in a hospital. They are true with everyone, including your own self-talk. You want to make sure that you are very real and sincere with yourself when you are being introspective. You want to make sure that you are able to put yourself in your own shoes. I know that sounds counter-intuitive, but it is important when you are trying to figure out why you did something in a certain way.

If you understand why you did something that you were not happy with, you will be able to forgive yourself. When you can do this, then you are ready to move to step three. This is to see what you need to do next and to show that you genuinely want the best for yourself. If you cannot step outside yourself to look and analyze the situation, then you're not going to be able to figure out the best course of action. You do not want to punish yourself for your bad behavior. You want to be able to disassociate your behavior from the essence of your being.

I conduct conferences on different ways to improve your self-talk. This is vital to be effective as a nurse because any negativity that you have will carry over to your work and be reflected back on to your patients. It will affect the communication between you and them. These three principles will always stay timeless and will always stand true. Remember them in this order: sincerity, empathy, and everyone is important. Let your patients and their families know that you genuinely want the best for them, and that you value them.

Conclusion

"Intelligence plus character; that is the goal of true education."

-Dr. Martin Luther King Jr.

We discussed the top three ways to increase patient satisfaction, which were communication, specifically nurse communication. Make sure that your communication is sublime and top notch. This is really the core thread in all surveys and interactions. It is what makes up the patient experience.

A way to increase patient satisfaction is responsiveness. When you communicate, do it with integrity. If you say you're going to do something, you do it when you say you will. You have to meet the patient's needs and satisfy them as quickly as possible.

Cleanliness is also important. You can have the greatest communication and be responsive, but it is important that you respect and value your environment. How the hospital looks reflects back on the patient and determines how he or she values and respects the hospital.

We also talked about the top three attitudes a nurse demonstrates at all times. First, is understanding. You have to be able to relate and to connect with the

patient. Then you need to be solution-orientated. Nurses are not complainers. If a
patent grumbles, offer a solution. A nurse
always has a positive outlook. Positivity
breeds positivity. By maintaining a positive
outlook and doing the best to see the good
in every situation, you can make sure the
patient experience is a great one.

Finally, we went over the top three
principles of what means the most to a patient. Above all else, a nurse has to be sincere. Keep it real, be honest and and stay
true. After that, a nurse needs to be em-
pathetic. They have to see things from the
other person's perspective. They have to
put themselves in that person's shoes and
to feel what they are feeling and see what
they are seeing. You can then relate and

connect on a deep level emotionally with the patient.

Last, but not least, is to make them feel important. Do this in everything that you do. Whether you are delivering pain meds, delivering a lifesaving operation, or just getting them water, make your patient feel important. Doing this is crucial in establishing a bond with the patient and can make all the difference in improving their experience at the hospital.

The goal of this book is to inspire you to think intensively about these attitudes and principles. You then need to evaluate how they relate to your character. After you do, I can promise you that you will be a much better person and a much better nurse.

About the Author

Daniel Truth Morgan's passion is to help nurses increase the connection they have with their patients. He believes that this is the key to a better experience for both the patient and nursing staff, and will lead to a better reputation for any hospital and medical staff that utilizes these principles.

Besides his practical experience as a nurse, Daniel is a Summa Cum Laude graduate of Stony Brook University with a Bachelor of Science in Nursing. Before that, he was a Summa Cum Laude graduate of Nassau Community College with associate degrees in both nursing and liberal arts. Not to mention, he is recipient of the prestigious SUNY Chancellor's Award.

In addition to nursing, Daniel is a life coach, trainer, and speaker. While he can certainly help a nursing staff optimally communicate with their patients, he has adapted these important concepts to any company or organization. To book Daniel to speak at your hospital or organization, call 631-392-8406 or email danieltruthmorgan@gmail.com

Made in United States
Orlando, FL
12 October 2022